Mindful

Wellbeing

A practical approach to a healthier, happier
and more contented life.

Vol 6

Extract from the original book,

'A Glimpse in a Transient Zone'

Jo Eaton.

Copyright.

Disclaimer.

The author of this book does not dispense medical advice or prescribe the use of any technique as a form of treatment for physical or medical problems without the advice of a physician, either directly or indirectly. The intent of the author is only to offer information of a general nature to help you in your quest for emotional and spiritual well-being. In the event you use any of the information in this book for yourself, which Is your constitutional right, the author and the publisher assume no responsibility for your actions.

In order to protect identity, I have changed the names of some of the characters within many of the stories.

Contents

Chapter 1

Connecting with the Energy in Nature

Energy is neither created or destroyed and as our soul is energy, it too cannot be destroyed, just always in a state of constantly changing, in harmony within the 'vast energy soup' of the Universe.

In order to attain your optimum health and wellbeing, it is important to raise your energy and vibration levels. It is better to live in the now, rather than the past or future, in the knowledge there is an infinite energy within the universe and so there is no limit to this energy and intelligence, no matter whatever your age.

It has been many years since I absorbed the concept of not being in isolation in this quantum soup, but feeling as an amoeba, vibrating clusters of energy, constantly changing, being ageless and eternal.

A way of enhancing your energy is to lose yourself in nature with forest walks, visiting gardens and the countryside, appreciating the beauty around you, always being drawn to loving and peaceful environments, rather than the lower energy field activities and conditions. This will intensify the feeling of wellbeing.

It has now been scientifically proven the healing properties of being in nature, with tree hugging increasing the hormone oxytocin, which induces a feeling of calm and emotional bonding. Also, released is serotonin and dopamine, which makes us feel much happier. Meanwhile, the earthy smell of the forest floor, releases phytoncides, which lower the heart rate, reduces blood pressure and boosts the immune system.

I think it is important to try to slow down and appreciate our surroundings, to listen to the birds, insects, falling rain and all the other endless sounds, smells and colours of nature, in all its beauty. We have so much to learn from this beautiful healing environment.

Another way to increase your energy level is through sound. Once again, it is important to be selective about the type of music you listen to because the negative lyrics, incorporating anger, fear, and violence, will deplete your energy. Whereas the sounds of nature, wonderful birdsong at Springtime in the forest or even beautiful tranquil music, full of positivity, love and peace, will also help raise your energy level.

It is not only energy fields but also sound waves are resonating from plant forms. In Damanhur, Turin, in northern Italy there are experiments taking place where sound recordings from plants have been recorded, noting that different plants make different sounds. This research has developed even further, whereby a recording has taken place of a vocalist, singing with the plants and as the music changed key, then the plants also changed their sound, in order to harmonise with the singer. I find this sort of communication of energies absolutely stunning. It proves we are all interconnected and part of this swirling energetic 'soup', in a state of flux. What a wonderful thought if a whole forest of plant forms were recorded and played alongside musicians.

From the above experiments, if we are so connected to nature's energy, then it is possible for our mental energy and thought process to have an effect on our natural surroundings. This method of communication is far more advantageous for the harmony of our planet because as humans, we presently manipulate each other to gain control through a psychological boost. This is most likely the reason of conflicts not only on a personal level but amongst other nations too.

Chapter 2

Increasing your Energy
from Food

Food is a way of gaining more energy, by chewing very slowly while appreciating and savouring the taste, in order to absorb the full value of the energy. As a result of this increased energy, you become more sensitive to surroundings and places that have this same heightened energy field. With practise, we are able to harness this energy from such environments. This method is so much more advantageous than the present fact of humans increasing their personal energy by psychologically taking it from others.

It is also important to take care of what type of food you put in your body. Our human form is a marvellous machine and so for the best performance, we need the best fuel in our 'tank', in order to allow our energy vibration to increase. I try to eat organic food whenever possible, to avoid any artificial additives, colourings, gluten and grains, which may have been sprayed with harmful pesticides. I have noticed my body will always let me know what foods I need to avoid. I am not a vegetarian but I only buy food with the animal welfare being paramount. Most of our fresh produce is sourced locally from a nearby farm. Trying to eliminate toxins from your food chain will also help your body maintain optimum health and so able to vibrate at a much higher level. One of the ways to increase our energy is to consume food since it contains stored sunlight which we need to expand our awareness, sharpen our concentration and further develop our senses. We need to eat more slowly too, to obtain the benefit from our food, to eat consciously and choose food which is fresh with vibrant colours. So many people today are distracted from the activity and pleasure our food gives us, by either watching television or using various media devices at mealtimes. This is such a shame and waste of valuable opportunity to increase our vibration.

From a personal experience, I have noticed after only a few days of eating an alkaline diet, my head feels so clear, as a starry night. I have clarity of thought and my perceptions and reactions are so much sharper. When I have eaten too much acid within my diet, I have had a problem with mobility and with eczema. Both problems disappear when I revert to a strict alkaline diet. I need to listen to my body, telling me what I need to eat. Through meditation, I became aware of not only eating a simple diet but also the importance of drinking lots of water, as this will assist the energy to resonate more easily within your body. In order to have a clear mind, it is essential to keep toxins out of your body, and this includes being careful or even withdrawing from alcohol, caffeine, artificial drugs and other low energy substances altogether.

Also, to take good care of our body by only eating good food, containing pure energy, carefully avoiding toxins too. Recently, my food intolerances have greatly increased, telling me to take notice so as my body becomes cleansed, then this allows for a higher resonance of energy, resulting in a stronger body.

By making conscious choices of the type of food we put into our body, allows us to maintain a higher level of vibration. This high level of energy will then flow outwards from your aura and into your environment. If everyone, collectively practised this way of life, then the whole consciousness of our planet would be raised to a higher, harmonious energy level. It is then, when the synchronistic processes are most active, so we must always stay alert for such happenings.

 Projecting this spiritual energy to others is beneficial for the well-being of everyone. It is the same when sending healing Reiki over long distances, where you become a channel to send vibrant, healing energy.

Chapter 3

Maintaining High Level of Energy

It is important to keep our body energy levels high, in order to attain optimum health benefits because there is a connection between low vibrations leading to stress and disease. It is good for our wellbeing to practise love and positive thoughts to keep us vibrating at the right level.

I am also aware that as part of this wellbeing, we need to maintain an enthusiasm for life, to look deeply within, to remember our life purpose, an insight into the future as to what we need to produce and it is this inspiration that keeps you young, vibrant, full of energy with positive thoughts. I know when I am on my right path because I feel so uplifted, full of joy and happiness. It just feels right, working on an intuitive level, while this state of excitement with life is extremely good for our own wellbeing and healing. It is working on this level, that I become more aware of synchronicity, of events and people entering my life, just at the right moment, in order to assist my endeavours. This is why it is so important to raise your energy level when it is depleted, in order that this flow continues to support your wellbeing and spiritual journey. I also note that more people are willing to talk about such matters, rather than in twenty or even ten years ago. I have noticed that in medicine, doctors are more readily prepared to listen and treat a patient in an holistic way, now being aware of the benefits of alternative therapies, as a treatment for prevention, rather than dismissing such theories. My own doctor thirty-five years ago, would not entertain such methods, but over time, she began to compromise and change her otherwise rigid views.

 I find it interesting to see this development around technology, where we are not only wanting information and liberation from mundane tasks, but we also are concerned about the effect upon our world. We want to attain an environmentally friendly technological existence which is finely attuned to our natural world. It is very important worldwide to achieve this delicate balance for the good health of ourselves and our planet.

Our brain patterns of thought also determines our wellbeing. For example, if we become depressed and introverted, then our energy vibrations are lowered, leaving us susceptible to disease. Therefore, it is important to raise our energy levels by taking an interest in life, in meeting people, travelling and learning new skills etc., to carry on growing, in order to retain an enthusiasm for life, resulting in higher energy, more vitality and a better healthy life style. We need to tell our bodies about our intentions, rather than expecting to decline with advancing years, because our body will follow our thought patterns. If we think old, then we grow old.

I believe our health problems are due to our low energy vibration, when we allow our senses to control our life. Change the way you see situations in your life, then the vibration increases and, as a result, good health returns.

I have just returned from a shopping trip to the supermarket where I observed a great majority of shoppers were living in a low energy field, their faces being drawn, no smiles, shoulders rounded, shuffling around like unhappy souls. If only they became aware of increasing their vibration, then their life would change for the better.

Obviously, if you are happy and feeling positive, then your body responds by being well and healthy. I have sometimes set out to openly smile to passers-by and maybe help a few elderly shoppers with their wears and it never ceases to impress me on how strangers are so grateful of such small actions. Their comments are very heart-warming and the rewards of the 'feel good factor' last for many hours. If only I could remember to operate on this level every day, instead of being within 'my own world'.

 It is through meditation that we are able to increase our energy, develop our intuition and creativity, so we are able to extend this knowledge and use this energy for the good of all. Breathing in this energy, allows us to elevate to a higher plane, so we need to adjust our actions accordingly, by living through positivity and unconditional love. As like attracts like, we need to aim high and create new, clear intentions and then believe your body will follow suit. I believe if you expect to live a long life, then your body will acknowledge this message, such is the power of expectation.

Some of my contemporaries are bored with life, with no forward plans and so their body follows this negative attitude and appears much older than their years. I guess their lives will be much shorter because of the depleted energy, lethargy and lack of enthusiasm and love for life. Anytime in our life, it is never too late to change our attitude, to create a new experience and in doing so, change our life.

We just need to look at setbacks or difficulties as lessons we need to learn on our journey. We need to concentrate on our aims, rather than what we do not have in life because this will attract more of what you do not want. I know I have a habit of whinging and complaining if things are not right, which is an expression of negativity. I have improved but I still have more work to do on my critical ego, always looking for perfection. I try to give thanks and express gratitude to those people in my life, but I know I need to extend this practise even further. Maybe it is a cultural thing but I do not find it easy to accept compliments or to express verbally how I feel emotionally about valued people in my life. I have often worked on the premise of actions speak louder than words, which was the environment I was brought up in, but generally, the social climate of to-day is very different, where people are encouraged to be more open and talk about their feelings. I try to send love, compliments, hugs and generous gestures and kindness most days, to those people in my life, for this generosity is not working through finances but working from the heart. It is an intuitive, spiritual way of interacting.

Chapter 4

Eradicating Fear and Releasing Negative Feelings

I believe we are here to learn, not suffer and that life is like a large classroom with numerous lessons and opportunities for us to experience. Through our relationships we have the opportunity to discard our negative traits of fear, anger, hatred etc and to develop the positive qualities of love, humility, kindness etc., while remembering to love ourselves too. I am so comforted to know our spiritual guides are always there to help us, sending love and support, while not expecting a reward or thanks. When we work on letting go of our negative habits, then this leads us to the cleansing of the true diamond within each of us.

Even members of our family are able to transfer their negative feeling towards others within the group. My own Mum used to relate her own family experiences at great length, some of which were very upsetting and although I was a young child at the time, I used to absorb those negative feelings. There is often a sadness disguised within our angry response. It is so important to try to understand the cause of this situation, letting go of this negativity, replacing it with love because being in a state of anger is very damaging for our bodies since, while in this state, we produce harmful chemicals that effect our heart, blood pressure, stomachs and immune systems, to name a few.

It was through meditation and the realisation that I was safe, loved and that nothing could really harm me or my spirit, that helped me to eradicate fear in my life. I know I am never alone and that all is well, because we are spiritual beings, in our physical bodies. If I find myself in a fearful situation, or if I actually absorb someone else's fear, then I try to withdraw from the situation and remind myself of my true origins. I am then immediately at peace, happy, calm and centred once again. This form of security will only come about through spirituality and not through material wealth. No one can ever take this sense of true protection away from you.

One important lesson I have learned throughout life's dramas is that nothing can really harm us because we are immortal, as we are spiritual beings having a human experience. I feel we are never alone as we each have our guardian spirits loving and taking care of us, so we need not be fearful of events or situations in our life, as this restricts our development. We are living out dramas as a means to increase our knowledge and intuition.

It is important to remember that this energy is very powerful, so if you reflect on negative past events in your life, this will result in a depletion of your energy and possible lead to illness. It is more beneficial for our good health to recognise our painful past life experiences, learn the lessons from them, then release them so energy is no longer drained from your body. Our energy system is similar to that of a battery. We need to keep it charged up, full of positive energy, in order to obtain the optimum performance.

We need to be mindful of circumstances or people who may reduce our energy. I call them 'energy suckers', the friends who are always 'needy', 'divas', insecure people, always wanting to absorb your energy, in order to make themselves feel better. A classic type of person is those with addictive personalities.   For example, drug addicts, smokers, gamblers, alcoholics etc. They are stuck on a circle of addiction, looking for support but often not heeding advice. I understand those types of personalities need help, but in doing so, it is important to protect and keep your own energy levels 'topped -up', otherwise, you too will have problems.

Throughout our development, we need to explore our character, to examine why we behave in the way we do with others, with addiction, with envy, with constant excuses, with shame etc. I call it 'soul searching' to examine our negative behaviour, then looking for the possible reasons, whether it maybe to do with our earlier life or past times, when such acts were adopted. Once the reasons for such behaviour is understood, then it is possible to change such habits into a more positive response.

This activity maybe very painful, to relive places in your childhood, where such ways of coping in certain circumstances were learned, just to survive at the time. Once this negative action is released, replaced by a new behaviour, generated by a loving, positive energy, then this is very cathartic way towards self-knowledge.

Caring for ourselves is very important, to release and forgive people for past demeanours, because in forgiving them, you are releasing the negative energy that may be harming yourself. Holding onto an old emotional wound just hurts yourself, not others and so hampers your progression.

Since anger and envy are negative emotions and linked to the ego, I try to cultivate unconditional love, incorporating a sense of peace and deeper meanings within my relationships, free from violence and rising above offensive comments. I have tried to live following those rules for more than thirty-five years, when I have never felt alone. This secure feeling, diminishes a sense of fear due to being aligned with the Source, allowing synchronistic events to occur.

It is also a good idea not to dwell on the past or to wish we had made different decisions on our journey through life. You are not going to be able to change the past and so it is a waste of time and accruing negative energy to live in regret. It is far better to learn from our mistakes and face the future with optimism, better equipped with this additional knowledge.

As I have realised that learning is remembering what we have forgotten, then teaching is reminding others that they know as much as you. If you want to remove an unwelcome incident or memory from your life, then just relax and remove it from your thoughts by using an imaginary eraser until the image within the clouds diminishes and it finally disappears. Another wisdom is when you are pulled, then you push, when you are pushed, then you pull. Those actions use the other persons strength against themselves, rather than against yourself.

One valuable lesson I have learned in life is to know when to push forward and when to hold back. Every now and again, it is useful to look into what is happening in your life, so you can have a sort of 'spring clean'. For example, I have re-examined past problems and blockages in my life so I can deal with them once and for all, so I may move on. If you are unable to resolve the problem, particularly if it involves another person, then it is best to release any negative feelings towards them and send them on their way, with love, so you may both heal and continue with your own journeys. In areas such as our relationships with both family, friends, our careers, emotional, physical etc., just let go so we may heal and then move onto better things with our increased vibration.

Chapter 5

Tranquil Spaces, while Limiting Excessive Use of Technology, Enhances Peace and Happiness

When aligning your creativity with Source, it is important for your intention to incorporate kindness as you follow your desired path. From research, it is known that serotonin, a naturally produced chemical in the brain, has a positive response to an act of kindness, not only for the giver, the recipient, but also to the observer of this act of kindness. Serotonin, not only improves the immune system, eases depression, but also gives the feeling of peace and happiness.

Making sure your home is clean and clutter free will ensure a positive environment in which to live. A peaceful, light, tranquil space, where there is room to attract an abundance within your life. Incorporate plants and fresh flowers which emit positive energy, colourful paintings, books, family photos full of fun memories and happy times, fragrance, spiritual areas, all add to this harmonious, peaceful ambiance.

I am also aware of the excessive use of technology, although I know it is a huge part of everyday life in the twenty-first century and almost impossible to totally avoid. I try not to use a computer for more than a few hours each day, and certainly not later than six hours before bedtime, otherwise

I have disturbed sleep. I limit the use of a mobile, the microwave, the TV and have the Wi-fi turned off at home, all in an attempt to restrict the exposure to low energy consumerism.

Now, I want peace and love in my life and I try to be loving, generous and kind towards myself and others each day. I still have to work on this task since I have a habit of pushing myself, never content with what I have achieved, but rather looking at the tasks I have been unable to complete. However, I reconcile myself with the idea I am always moving forward, not at the quicker pace I would have liked, but with life's endless interruptions, I must settle for my best efforts. This, I resolve, is being kind to myself. I know we are all worthy of the abundance in the universe and there is plenty of positive energy to go around for all of us.

Chapter 6

Radiating Positive Energy

By raising your own energy field and controlling your ego, then everyone you meet will be affected by your energy field, as ripples in a pool. Each and every one will benefit from this positive energy that emits from you and others, connecting us to our Source while assisting us towards our desires and destiny.

Over the years when teaching, I have become aware that I am totally absorbed into my subject, when trying to put a point across, so I totally forget about self and ego. This enthusiasm, in turn, happens to transfer onto the students, leaving them energized, without imparting any words. I realise this vitality translates through your presence. However, if you constantly manipulate conversations as an opportunity to talk about self, then this is an ego-driven low energy activity, which will be detrimental to the progression of others, leaving them with a feeling of low self-esteem. If you are connected to the universal energy, staying focused on creating a loving and positive energy field, this mode of working promotes a healthy immune system and good health. You become too busy to give ill health any energy or attention. It is important to maintain this stimulating presence for the benefit of all as the higher vibrating energy will help counterbalance any negative energy.

Another way of enhancing your energy is to associate with like-minded friends and family, who radiate positive higher energy, to help others with acts of kindness, while never looking for praise or repayment

As I have journeyed through life, I have realised the importance of healing self and in doing so, to help others too. By thinking positive thoughts and forward thinking to times when you felt very well, when at the time you are not feeling so good, then your energy raises and your body remembers that positive healthy state and will help you to return to good health, to restore your body to correspond to the energy of your thoughts.

Our physical body is surrounded by energy too. The aura extends about a metre from the body, in most people and yet it is possible to enlarge your aura even further through development and meditation. Sometimes, it is noticeable for someone to enter a room and the whole area 'lights up'. The complete ambience of the room changes in a good way. This is usually due to our sensitive auras constantly transmitting and receiving sublime messages to us about our environment. Obviously, the opposite may also happen if someone who is experiencing some difficulties in their life. when they enter the room, the whole dynamics of the room will have a depletion of energy.

This energy aura is a good indicator of our wellbeing, because before we become physically ill, our body's energy diminishes and so loses its vitality. This is an indicator for us to change our actions or way of thinking, in order to promote self-healing. This is our natural way of a warning, so if we do not change our actions, then the next step our body takes is for us to be physically ill. Usually this is a stark warning for us not to ignore the messages and correct what is causing a problem in our life, because we need to maintain a supply of positive energy within our body and aura, to stay in good health. When you come across like-minded people, there is an instant recognition, 'a knowing'. It is very difficult to explain, but each are aware of there being 'something'.

Living from a higher self may start with small adjustments like when you maybe in a conversation with a friend and they are being driven by their ego. It is better to recognise this and not counter intervene with another ego statement, but rather stay quiet, or in agreement with them. Since this is a conscious decision, to avoid the lower energy interplay, then you are working in a higher energy field. Just refuse to be drawn in and not accept any negative comments intended for you. It is their Kama and so better not to clash, taking an opposite stance.

 It is so easy to become drawn into this negative drama, particularly if everyone you speak to has a tale of woe. I try to privately wish them love and withdraw from the situation. This also happens if I find myself in the company of noisy adults, or even disruptive children, who are being ignored by their parents. I find those negative vibrations extremely upsetting, maybe more so, as my hearing has become even more acute, together with my other finely tuned senses.   Polluted food, noise and air pollution contribute to this low energy field. Once again, I find the best strategy is to privately ask for protection, then send my love, before moving from the low energy atmosphere.

It is so easy to be influenced by others too, if they are restless and wish to change job or home etc. You need to concentrate on what is good for you and yours, while staying focused on your journey, because if you are in a state of unease about your life and do not sort out the problem, then your physical body will become unwell.

In the book 'Illusions' by Richard Bach, I just love this quote:
'Don't be dismayed at goodbyes. A farewell is necessary before you can meet again. And meeting again, after moments or lifetimes, is certain for those who are friends.'

Chapter 7
Respecting your Body and Having Faith in Yourself

Looking after yourself by commencing a regular exercise regime and taking a pride in your appearance, is a way of respecting your body, leading to a more positive, optimistic attitude to life, while always envisaging yourself as being in good health, because your body will then follow suit. If you are pessimistic and depressed, then your body becomes depleted of energy and so illness follows. When I feel good, my energy field is high and I then feel full of enthusiasm to work on my creative projects, which in turn, makes me feel exhilarated. This circle of good feelings, just keeps spiralling as your positive energy increases.

I find it interesting to know that the skin replaces itself once each month, the stomach lining every five days, the liver every six weeks and the skeleton every three months and so by the end of a year, ninety-eight percent of the body would have been renewed. Throughout this change, intelligence, energy and information have been transferred to the new cells.

There are cases of people having received an organ transplant, who later became aware of a slight change in their behaviour, representing that of their donor. This appears to suggest a transference of intelligence.

I try to be active in my life, because this generates energy and a feeling of wellbeing. I am then in a position where I may help others, rather than needing others or trying to impress and gaining their approval. I suppose this attitude has been furnished by my sense of being so independent. I never realised just how driven and determined I was, until I had an accident and ended up in plaster. To have to rely on the help of other people was a new experience for me and so frustrating. I swiftly sorted out a way of being mobile again, under my own steam. Even returning to work on crutches. This was not driven by ego, but to look at the problem as a hindrance and by ignoring the situation, was my way of dealing with the injury independently.

However, although I am extremely focused on my intentions, I am still aware I am able to release and remove this project at any time. This concept maybe applied to relationships too because no one is indispensable. No one should have so much control over you so that you feel you are unable to walk away. This is giving your power away, a thing you should never do. You need to be together because you want to be, not because you need to be. There is a difference. You are able to love someone while not having to relinquish part of self too. That way, you will earn the respect of your partner.

Also be aware that all of us are constantly changing in this cosmic soup and so are the dynamics of our relationships, so it is always wise to need nothing from anyone. This is why I try to be self-sufficient and independent.

It is important too, that we focus on abundance, rather than on scarcity, because wherever you concentrate your energy, it magnifies and comes to fruition. For example, if you feel ill, then keep talking and thinking about it, then those feelings increase and so your illness becomes more severe. This is because you have given the problem more energy and attention. However, if you ignore the problem, letting your body do its job of healing, you are able to concentrate on the healthier parts of your body, so your energy follows suit and your recovery is much quicker.

There is no limit to this energy within our Universe. There is plenty to go around. I have noticed a large portion of my time in the past was spent on scarcity, what I did not have in my life, not enough money, not enough time, being upset if I had not completed my tasks for the day, rather than congratulating myself on how much I had completed. It is important to think of a glass half full, rather than half empty. I realised when teaching, if a student is working well, then by offering encouragement, that focus would grow, resulting in success. By shifting the focus from concentrating on what is missing in another person, but instead, concentrate on what you love about that person, then that positive emotion within the relationship increases.

Having faith in yourself is very important, when not taking external advice from others but to listen to your body. Your body's instinct will know what food you need to have, when you need to sleep, help itself or how to exercise etc. It maybe through dance, running or through other sports. Your body has the ability to follow its own wisdom. We just need to have faith and trust in this body instinct, because we can achieve far higher levels than we ever imagined. I know I am far stronger mentally than I ever thought possible.

Our brain is able to access higher wisdom, almost like an electronic antenna, drawing upon the universal intelligence. Due to this system, we each have everything we need. Our journey begins and ends with us and so any teacher in our life, is just assisting us to unlock our own potential, a vehicle of support, just to help us realise our true self. It is so very important to look after and respect self because we each have so much treasure, wisdom and knowledge locked within.

It is good to be kind to self too, allowing a few treats and luxuries because you too deserve to be treated well. We are all part of this changing universe, so it is pointless hoarding your possessions because all things are in transition. We are just temporary custodians for the short time we are here, so release the need to hold onto things, release the fear and be free.

For our wellbeing, I believe it is important to participate in pastimes which give us joy, as when dancing, walking in nature or creative ventures etc., for such activities are very similar to meditation and so need to be encouraged and nurtured as part of our daily routine. As I understand certain lessons along my way, it is like collecting pieces of a grand jigsaw, or even as a flower, with its petals slowly opening, before coming into full bloom.

Each day I look for a 'gift' or lessons to help me and others on our way, giving love, hugs, flowers, encouragement or time to listen to friends or strangers. Only this morning, the wind was blowing a gale and the rain was torrential, when I saw an elderly lady struggling with her shopping while trying to fasten her rain-hat. I went over to help her, fastening her hat securely under her chin. Only as I looked closely into the warm smiling face of the pensioner, did I realise it was someone who I recognised from more than thirty years earlier. What a lovely surprise and delight as we exchanged our news.

I know my circle seems to becoming even wider, attracting similar souls. I am more open about my intentions too, wishing to send love out into the world and with this increased sensitivity, I find it easier to tune into other peoples' emotions, knowing if they need a hug, a surprise gift to raise their spirits or whether it be due to loneliness or despair. With friends, neighbours and relatives, experiencing difficulties with life's lessons, it is a balancing act to maintain my own energy system, so it is quicker and easier to send telepathic messages. Also bearing in mind, this maybe a two-way exchange of supporting each other.

With passing time, I think we all begin to know ourselves very well, our strengths and our weaknesses. One of the first things I needed to do when I embarked on my Master's degree course, as a mature student, was to explain to my tutor, the way to get the best out of me, not to push for work because I am naturally extremely driven and will not miss deadlines, for him to be clear on what is expected of me and for me to be able to take control of my work. This first tutorial set down a solid foundation for the rest of the course. In fact, as it transpired, it was a two-way exchange, with me being able to help him with his personal problems too. However, this person did not feel a total stranger since he was someone I instantly recognised as a dear friend of mine from past-times, when I think I was a male friend at the time. He too believes there is something, but he is not quite sure what it is, yet even to this day, this friendship has still survived the test of time.

Gratitude

It is very important to practise gratitude and yet in our busy lives, it is so easy to forget to give thanks. One of my journals has been dedicated to our daily blessings, by just taking a few minutes at the end of each day to make a short list of the occasions during that time which you feel you need to express gratitude. It maybe how well you feel, or the beauty of the flowers on your windowsill, or possibly the warmth of a child's smile etc. This small activity helps us concentrate on regularly appreciating the blessings and love in our lives. At times, I have woken up at dawn, then watched the sun rise, the wonders of the changing hues of purples, pinks, delicate oranges turning to lucid yellows in the sky. The exquisite sound of peace, except for the harmonious chorus of bird song, the fragrance of the May blossom hanging heavy in the air. This is such a moving, almost spiritual experience, which reminds us of our connection with our very essence. My Grandma used to rise as the sun was appearing, to marvel at the serenity of this time of day, just as the vibration in nature is rising too.

Chapter 8

Reducing Stress by Introducing Structure in your Life

Making a habit of regularly checking our energy system is very important. For example, if there is stress in your life, then this must be addressed or if there is some other person who is reducing your energy, then look for the lesson which this 'teacher' is presenting to you, so you may learn from those actions of fear or blame. If you do not adjust your actions, then the lesson will continue to reoccur in some other form, until you have learned and then you become free to move on. Action heals rather than talking, but healing your body or dealing with life's challenges need to be addressed on a daily basis.

<u>Cosmic Ordering</u>.

As I have moved through my life, I have realised our negative thoughts hamper our progression. So, many years ago, I wrote a long list of those negative thoughts, almost surprising myself about what I wrote down. For example, lack of financial security, not being content with the place where I am living, being fearful of the changes ahead when embarking on a new job etc. I then set out and wrote about a whole new positive scenario, one which addressed and cancelled those negative thoughts, concluding the account with the following statement: ' This or something better is now manifesting for me in a totally satisfying and harmonious way, for the highest good of all concerned.' I then signed this statement with the intention of sending out my request into the universe, almost like placing an order.

Now, looking back at my negative list, some twenty-five years later, most of those comments have been cancelled out by some wonderful positive happenings in my life. There are but a few to materialise, yet I am still working towards those goals. So, my advice to you, is to list your negative thoughts which maybe holding you back from realising your potential, then write up an ideal scenario, full of your dreams and desires. Once signed, then trust and pass over the task to the universe and see what comes to fruition.

We need to learn to make a list of our desires and then just trust the Universe to connect you with whatever is necessary in your life. You create your thoughts, as energetic instructions and then actions will follow them. As we are each Divine being, full of great creative, intelligent potential, our energetic passion to create, transposes into reality. I believe this is how the creative process works.

Our requests may not be fulfilled immediately but then it is our duty to be patient and wait for our wishes to materialise. Sometimes, it is not always what we want which is the best option for us, as we are not privy to seeing the whole picture from our position. It maybe years down the line when you reflect on the past, then all becomes clear and most often events have worked out for the best.

I find the more you write down, whether it be your thoughts, aims, observations, spiritual happenings, evaluating your progress etc., then this exercise makes it easier to process the details, hence my numerous journals. It is good to have 'time out' too, when you need to store up your energy before advancing forward onto your next venture. I have had several years when I have not physically produced any artwork and yet my head has been processing certain ideas and themes. Instead, I have been consolidating my thoughts while 'resting', in the knowledge that all is well, as there are reasons for everything and along our way, we will be confronted with opportunities and obstacles as planned, before we were born.

I have been saddened and disappointed at not realising my dreams with my artwork, because I have a fear of wasting my gifts, at not being able to serve by using my honed skills to pass on knowledge. However, if it is meant to be, then it will happen, but in the meantime, I am writing a book, in the hope of servitude.

To feel secure in life is a spiritual trait, not an earthly one, so security can only come from within.

I find it very useful to annually make a plan for all areas of your life and so by setting goals, then seeing them written down on paper, you are then able to slowly move forward in achieving your aims. For example, I have made plans for where I would like to be in five years' time, four, three, two and one year, in the areas of my career, professional development, finances, relationships, household etc. If after a year, you have changed your mind about your goals, then that is fine, you have not failed. Just make the necessary adjustments, then review your progress annually, so you will have an overview of your progress. Make your affirmations clear, short and with strong convictions, setting out what you really want from life. I have always found this method of organisation very helpful and it has given me direction to my life, rather than wasting my time.

<u>Health and Food.</u>

Here are a few suggestions to help reduce your stress levels:

- As mentioned in the earlier chapter relating to 'Healing', there is meditation breathing exercises, while to calm nerves, just stroke the back of your left hand, very gently, with the palm of the right hand.
- With the tips of the first three fingers on the right hand, stroke the fingers on the left hand.
- Hands receive and transmit different waves and currents and what I always find intriguing is that I am able to identify the hands of family, friends and colleagues, in the same way as looking at their faces.
- When outdoors in nature, raise your hands in greeting to increase the bond between you and the Source, evident in the natural world. This increases your strength and light, so in turn, you pour out love and immediately this vacuum fills up again. With this work on your psychic image, after a while, your physical self will both become as one.

As we become more gentle, harmonious and peaceful, it is wise to continue working towards the highest ideal, in the knowledge it will always be out of reach, but our aim is to be the best we can be.

Since we are consciously participating in our evolving process, we always appear to attract those people and situations that we most need to further our development in this domain. We are responsible for our own healing, just as we are the sole initiator of our dramas and circumstances.

Energy lines.

Meridian lines are energy paths which conduct life force around the body, so it is important to keep them free because blocked energy cannot vibrate at the full optimum. Therefore, exercising, walking, dancing etc., will free the energy blockages and so increase your wellbeing.

Chapter 9

Conclusion

It is important to listen to our intuition, to listen to our body because if you have a health problem, your vibrating energy is not at its optimum. It is a good idea to frequently participate in activities to raise your vibration, which in turn will attract positive emotions and good health.

When I am preparing to create some artwork, as my enthusiasm increases, so does my vibrations, just ready to be released as I start work. My art returns me to my natural frequency. This I noticed when I was in mourning over the death of my Mum. I was healed by returning to my painting. The activity is almost like when meditating.

Sound and other ventures can also restore your energy balance, as it resonates with our cells and organs in our body. Also, controlled breathing, as when meditating, helps to heal problem areas of the body, by focusing on the positive energy travelling around until it releases any negative blocks that maybe causing a problem.

For a few minutes every day, focus on your aims for the future, then imagine in great detail, as if your dreams have already arrived. This activity, on a regular basis, will attract that particular energy into your life.

So, there are many ways in which you are able to improve your Well-Being; to eat healthily, meditate regularly to increase your vibrations and vitality, avoid excessive use of technology, focus on positive thoughts, exercise regularly and immerse yourself in the natural environment. Most importantly, learn to love yourself, love life and have fun.